10/98

Everything You Need to Know About

MONONUCLEOSIS

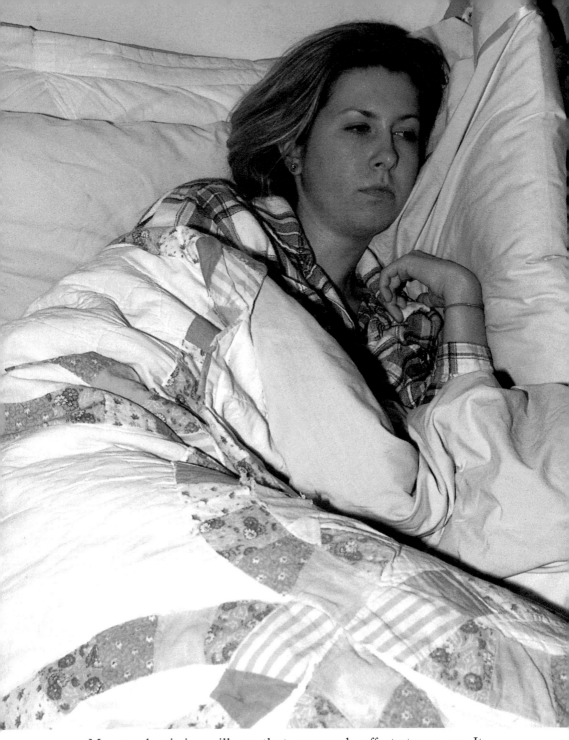

Mononucleosis is an illness that commonly affects teenagers. It tends to make people extremely tired, forcing them to stay home and rest until it has run its course.

Everything You Need to Know About

MONONUCLEOSIS

Paul Smart

THE ROSEN PUBLISHING GROUP, INC.
NEW YORK

Published in 1998 by The Rosen Publishing Group, Inc.
29 East 21st Street, New York, NY 10010

First Edition

Library of Congress Cataloging-in-Publication Data

Smart, P. (Paul), 1957-
    Everything you need to know about mononucleosis / Paul Smart. —
1st ed.
        p.   cm. — (Need to know library)
    Includes bibliographical references and index.
    Summary: Discusses the nature and diagnosis of mononucleosis and how to
protect against it or cope with having it.
    ISBN 0-8239-2550-1
    1. Mononucleosis—Juvenile literature.   [1. Mononucleosis. 2. Diseases.]
I. Title. II. Series.
RC147.G6S585   1998
616. 9'25--dc21   98-10119
                                                CIP
                                                 AC

Manufactured in the United States of America

Contents

Introduction

nnie was a high school junior. She was enjoying some of her classes, playing volleyball on the team, and starting to get calls for dates.

One morning, Annie woke up with a sore throat. From that day on, she felt tired all the time. Her eyes itched constantly, and she lost her appetite.

After a week, her symptoms still hadn't gone away. Annie's mom grew concerned and told her to stay home from school. Annie rested, but she didn't feel any better. She felt too tired to read or even to watch television. One night she found herself lying on the floor of the living room unable to move. She was too tired to ask for help or explain how bad she felt. She grew embarrassed about her strange illness and became deeply depressed about what was happening to her. It seemed as if she would never get better. What could be wrong with her?

After another week of feeling more and more tired, Annie's parents went with her to see the family doctor. The doctor ran some tests and determined that Annie had mononucleosis. He explained that the disease, quite common among teenagers, would run its course after several weeks.

He told Annie that there was no medicine to cure it. She would just have to take care of herself by getting plenty of rest, eating well, and drinking lots of liquids. And the doctor added that when she started feeling better, which would eventually happen, Annie would have to take it easy and not do anything too strenuous for at least a month following her bout with the illness.

Mononucleosis is a disease that usually strikes teens. Among teenagers, it is commonly known as the "kissing disease," the "sleeping disease," and "mono."

The only real cure for mononucleosis is rest. No known medications treat it effectively, except for helping to reduce the discomfort of specific symptoms. Sore throat, fever, loss of appetite, and fatigue are some of the many symptoms associated with mononucleosis.

Doctors say that the best method of coping with mononucleosis is to take care of yourself by getting plenty of rest, eating well, and drinking lots of beverages. Some suggest vitamins and the use of special over-the-counter remedies.

This book will help you understand mononucleosis so that you will know what precautions you can take to

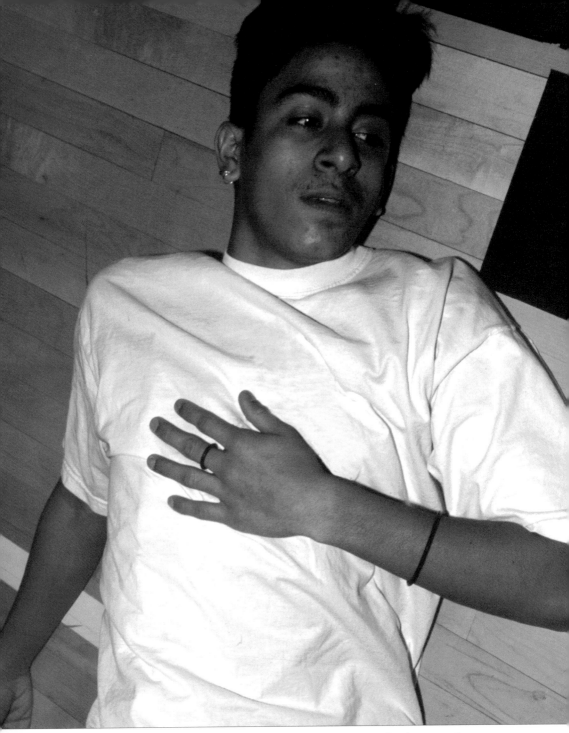

Someone who has mononucleosis may feel too tired or weak to perform tasks that otherwise require little effort, such as watching TV or getting out of bed.

avoid contracting it and how to take care of yourself if you do get it.

This book discusses what mononucleosis is and its symptoms. It also discusses the origin of the disease, current medical research, and what to do if you think you may have mononucleosis. It examines some theories about when and why mononucleosis tends to occur. Finally, the book discusses some preventive measures, things you can do to avoid getting mononucleosis.

As Annie found out, one of the worst aspects of mononucleosis is the suddenness with which it occurs and the depression it can cause in someone who has it. Mononucleosis can be much more serious than its nicknames imply.

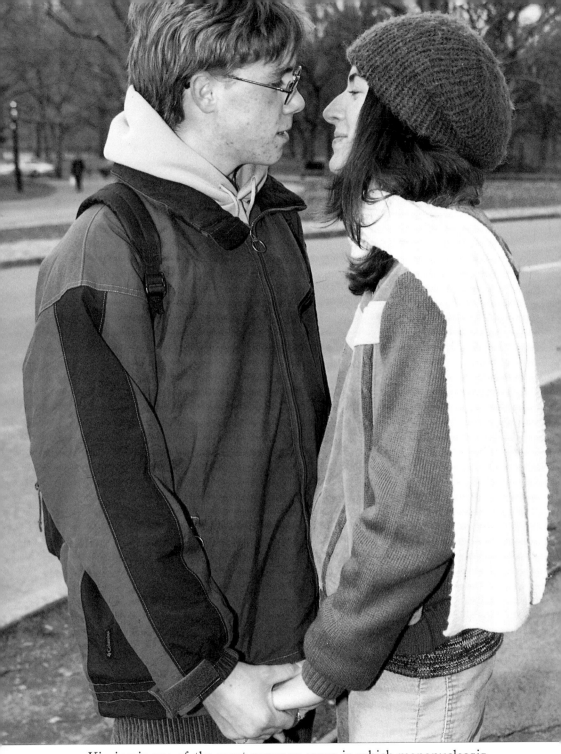

Kissing is one of the most common ways in which mononucleosis is spread.

Chapter 1

What Is Mononucleosis?

Mononucleosis is a contagious disease that is most common among people between the ages of fifteen and twenty-five. Medically, it's known as a variety of the Epstein-Barr virus. This means it is a type of herpes. The first cases of mononucleosis were identified in the 1920s.

"The Kissing Disease"

Mononucleosis is known as "the kissing disease," because kissing is one of the more common ways in which it is spread. Like most herpes-related viruses, it can be contracted, or caught, through oral or sexual contact.

The first case to come under close medical scrutiny occurred during the 1950s. It involved a number of West Point Army cadets. Their only shared experience was a train ride from New York City. Also on the train was a group of young women. All of the cadets who caught the disease admitted to having kissed one of the women in this group.

Mononucleosis is also known as "the sleeping disease" because it makes a person very tired. Doing anything becomes a big effort. Even small activities, such as watching television or reading a book, can tire someone with mono.

People with mononucleosis can have symptoms ranging from mild to severe. It varies from person to person. One of the worrisome things about a disease like mononucleosis is how little is known about it. It is comforting that it goes away by itself, and that it almost never occurs a second time. But why does it go away, and what causes it to develop in the first place?

Immunology

Although people have been suffering from mono for a long time, scientists still don't know that much about it. Immunology, the study of the immune system, is a growing field and may be able to provide the answers scientists have been looking for.

The questions of how the immune system works and how it can be damaged or weakened are now receiving a great deal of attention from the medical community. The appearance and spread of the human immunodeficiency virus (HIV), and of acquired immunodeficiency syndrome (AIDS), an often fatal sexually transmitted disease (STD), has prompted a greater interest in the study of immunology.

HIV attacks the immune system, and eventually destroys it. This leaves the body vulnerable to disease. Even diseases that are usually harmless to a person whose immune system is working properly can kill a person with a weakened immune system. Although there is treatment to help extend the lives of people who are HIV-positive (those who test positive for HIV), there is still no cure.

In the goal to find a cure for AIDS, doctors and scientists are doing research on other illnesses involving the immune system. This includes Epstein-Barr virus and mononucleosis. Work is under way to find ways of keeping people from catching mononucleosis and helping people recover from it more quickly once they have it.

What Doctors Say

In medical terms, mono is called a "self-limiting viral disease" with "nonspecific symptoms." Viral disease means that the disease is passed from one person to another in the form of a virus, similar to that of a cold. It is self-limiting because a person catches it once and his or her body becomes immune to it. Nonspecific symptoms means that all of the symptoms that characterize mononucleosis also characterize other ailments. Only medical tests can determine whether symptoms are the result of mono or just a bad cold.

The Immune System

The immune system is made up of blood cells; attack proteins, such as antibodies, that help fight infections; and organs, including the thymus, spleen, lymph nodes, and bone marrow. These different parts work together to battle threats, such as viruses and other germs, which can damage the body. The immune system also works by preventing them from becoming serious threats to the body. When a harmful bacterium or virus enters the body, the immune system goes into action to try to destroy it.

Even the smallest changes in the immune system can weaken it, allowing a person to "catch" diseases, such as mononucleosis. Although researchers continue to investigate what causes an immune system to weaken, they don't have all the answers.

How the Immune System Works

When a harmful bacterium, virus, or other germ enters the body, the immune system goes into action to destroy it. A cut in the skin, for instance, can allow germs to enter. In the case of mononucleosis, the virus is usually spread through saliva. Once the body is infected, the immune system goes to work.

The first response of the immune system is found in the blood. Two classes of white blood cells rush to the site of an intruding germ and try to destroy it. One class of white blood cells, called macrophages, engulf most foreign particles and digest them. The other class of

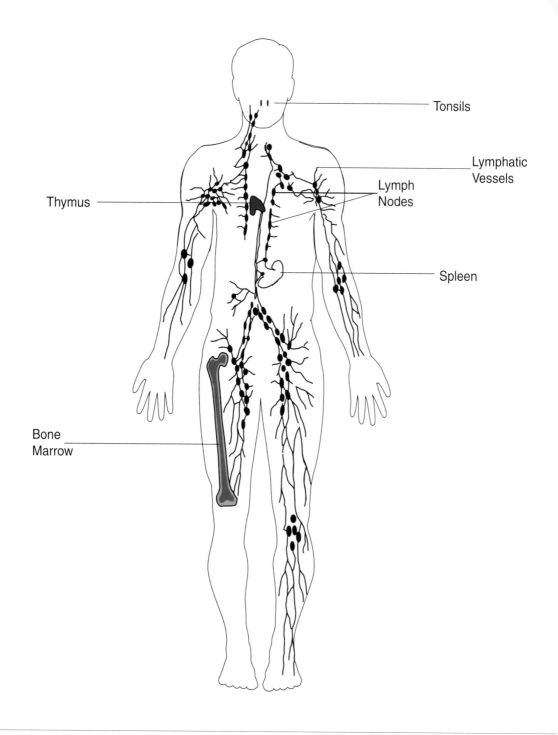

Tonsils

Lymphatic
Vessels

Thymus

Lymph
Nodes

Spleen

Bone
Marrow

The immune system is made up of various organs and bodily
systems that work together to protect the body from germs that
cause illnesses.

white blood cells, called lymphocytes, release attack proteins which bind to and kill the intruding germ.

The second response of the immune system involves the lymphatic system. The lymphatic system fights germs that enter the body by serving as a filter system for the body's other cells. It consists of a set of vessels that drains excess fluid, called lymph, from the body's cells.

At various sites in the body, the lymphatic vessels connect to lymph nodes, which act as checkpoints that filter out particles from the lymph fluid and produce other cells of the immune system. Lymph nodes also serve to maintain a balanced distribution of lymph fluid in the body. They are located in the neck, groin, and armpits. The tonsils, for example, are lymph nodes in the neck.

The spleen is a large mass of lymphatic tissue that produces new blood cells and filters out impurities from the bloodstream. The spleen also stores fresh blood for use if the body goes into sudden shock.

The thymus is one of the body's main glands of the immune system. It produces a class of white blood cells, called T cell lymphocytes, that can destroy an intruding germ or virus by releasing attack proteins. The T cells also act to regulate the responses of the other cells of the immune system.

Bone marrow inside your bones contains the beginnings of all types of cells found in the blood. In addition, bone marrow produces lymphocytes called B cells.

These lymphocytes release the attack proteins called antibodies, which kill invading germs or viruses. Once antibodies are produced and released by B cells during an infection, they remain in the body to help fight off new infections.

All of these parts of the immune system work together to protect the body against invaders.

What Does It Mean to Be Immune?

Once a person has had mononucleosis, he or she cannot contract it again. He or she has become immune to it. The person's immune system has developed antibodies that can kill the virus. The body also remembers the virus, so that if it enters the body again, the body immediately releases the antibodies to destroy it.

However, the best protection against illness and disease is to keep the immune system strong and healthy. This involves maintaining the right nutritional balance through proper eating habits, vitamin intake, exercise, and rest.

Doctors are finding that once the immune system has been damaged, as happens with AIDS and similar diseases, the body is no longer able to fight disease as efficiently as it once had.

Although a person will not get mono twice, other forms of the Epstein-Barr virus can enter the body. They can cause other illnesses very similar to mono, such as chronic fatigue syndrome (CFS). CFS will be discussed in more detail in chapter 3.

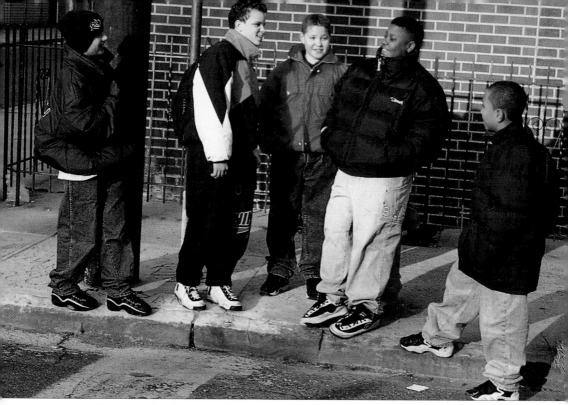
Mononucleosis can strike anyone.

The Epstein-Barr Virus

Viruses cause infectious diseases. Infections are diseases that can be spread to others. Mononucleosis is an infectious disease caused by a type of herpes virus called the Epstein-Barr virus.

Herpes viruses are a group of viruses that cause diseases involving inflammation of the skin and breakdowns in the lymph system. These diseases include chicken pox, cold sores, fever blisters, herpes simplex, and mononucleosis.

The Epstein-Barr virus was first identified in children from Africa who were suffering from a type of cancer known as Burkitt's lymphoma. This disease causes the lymph nodes to swell.

Researchers later found that the Epstein-Barr virus primarily attacks the lymph system, which is part of the immune system. Once the lymph system is weakened, a person fighting the Epstein-Barr virus is more susceptible than usual to other illnesses. The immune system is not able to fight off other illnesses as efficiently.

Doctors are unsure of exactly how the Epstein-Barr virus causes mononucleosis. They do know that the virus is present in all cases of mono. They are still unsure what other diseases the virus causes.

Doctors also know that mono usually strikes the immune system. Glands will swell. The tonsils will hurt. The skin will feel hot and stretched out. All of these symptoms may cause a person to have greater fatigue than do other illnesses. Because mono causes symptoms in many parts of the immune system, the body tires out quickly.

Why Me?

According to experts, 90 percent of all adults have somehow contracted and developed an immunity to the Epstein-Barr virus at some time in their lives. They know this because antibodies and traces of the virus itself show up in the white blood cell counts when adults are tested for viral diseases.

Ninety percent of teens do not catch mononucleosis. So how did 90 percent of adults get exposed to the Epstein-Barr virus that causes mononucleosis without becoming infected? Aside from the few cases of Burkitt's lymphoma uncovered in Africa, the Epstein-

Barr virus does not show up anywhere else. It is, however, suspected as a cause of chronic fatigue syndrome, a disease still in the early stages of being studied.

Mononucleosis and Childhood

Most people catch the virus and develop immunity to mononucleosis during childhood. The reason most people, including doctors, don't notice that children have mono is because its symptoms are similar to those of a lot of other illnesses. Most parents probably assume their child has a cold or the flu. And in some ways, children are in a better position to fight such diseases than are teens and young adults.

Children tend to go to bed earlier and get more rest, which helps to keep the immune system strong. Children also do not face many of the problems that teens do. Most children fight mononucleosis more easily than do teens, because children don't have to worry as much about juggling homework, a job, after-school sports, a social life, or some combination of those demands. Such commitments often take their toll on the immune system because of the level of stress they produce.

Those who do not contract mononucleosis during childhood will often develop it during their teen years. This can be difficult because the disease often forces the teens to slow down. Because of their busy schedule of school, friends, and work, some teens find it hard to slow down. It is often harder for them to find the time to rest.

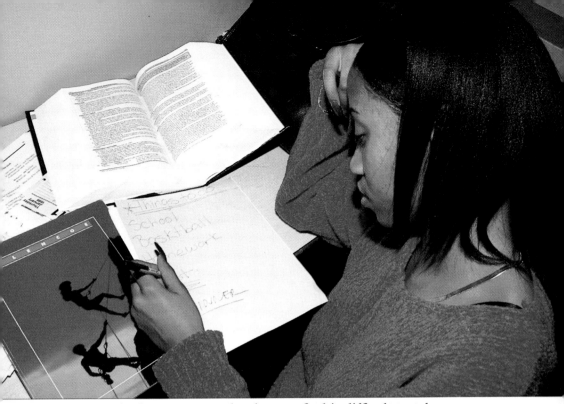

Teens who have mononucleosis may find it difficult to take a break from their busy schedules and take time to rest.

Patience is one of the keys to helping the body repair itself. But for an active teen, it may be difficult to slow down. That is why the disease is sometimes accompanied by bouts with mental, as opposed to clinical, depression, which in turn makes it harder for the body to get well.

Mononucleosis occurs more frequently in young women than in young men. This is apparently because boys tend to play more roughly and physically with each other than do girls. Because of the close physical contact, the Epstein-Barr virus can be easily passed through saliva. Many boys may have contracted mono and become immune to it during childhood. Likewise, recent research has shown that children who don't play much

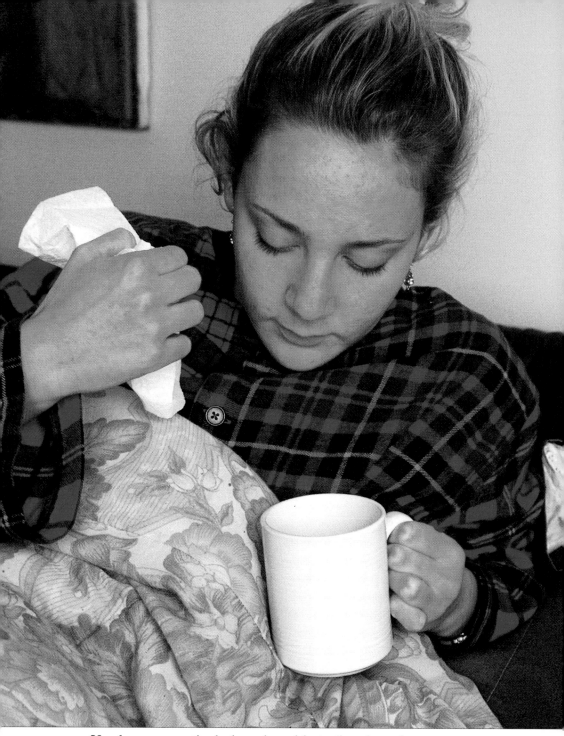

You become particularly vulnerable to the virus that causes mononucleosis when your immune system is weakened by another illness, such as the flu.

with other children their age have less opportunity to catch the disease during childhood.

Teenagers often contract mono during the exchange of saliva through kissing. It appears that teens sometimes become infected with mono because something else has affected their immune system. A cold, the flu, an allergy, or emotional stress can weaken the body. A weakened immune system can allow a virus to get past its defenses.

Chapter 2

Symptoms

Time is the one thing necessary to recover from mononucleosis. Mono takes between one and two months to work its way through the body. Full recovery can take an additional two to four months.

It is important to remember that the symptoms of a disease are its result and not its cause. When you catch mononucleosis, you get tired because of the disease. Similarly, you get a sore throat, decreased appetite, and maybe a rash because you are sick. This is one way your body protects itself: It corners an illness in certain areas of the body where it can best fight it.

What Are the Symptoms?

Whether mild or severe, symptoms of mononucleosis are uncomfortable. People with mild cases of mononucleosis may exhibit only a few symptoms. People with

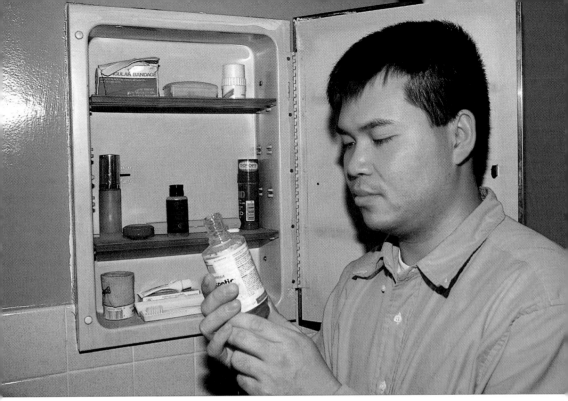

While no medicine can cure mononucleosis, your doctor can prescribe certain medications to relieve your symptoms.

more severe cases may exhibit most or all symptoms. Common symptoms include:

- fever
- dehydration
- fatigue
- runny nose
- sore throat
- loss of appetite
- nausea
- swollen glands

Rosa

Rosa contracted mono during the finals of her junior

*year in high school. She had a great job lined up for sum-
mer vacation. She was more than ready to relax for a
while after working hard to try to keep her grades up.
She had had her ups and downs all year at school, but
the school year was almost over, and she was looking
forward to the summer.*

*When Rosa started feeling tired, she thought it was
because of the stress from studying. She promised herself that she would relax once the school year was over.
She had so many things to do before the summer.
Although she had already taken most of her finals, she
still had a couple left. She was planning to go to the graduation to see some of her friends graduate. She was also
invited to a few graduation parties. But after a couple
of weeks, she felt so ill that she decided to see her doctor. He ran some tests, including a blood test. The doctor diagnosed Rosa with mononucleosis.*

*Rosa had to miss her friends' graduations, all of the
parties at the end of the school year, and a couple of her
finals. And she had to cancel her summer job plans in
order to stay home so she could get well.*

How Do I Know It's Mononucleosis?

Health specialists suggest that the best way of checking whether you have this disease is to start by treating
individual symptoms. Following are some suggestions
on how to treat the symptoms.

Generally, if your symptoms go away within a day
or two, you do not have mononucleosis. If symptoms

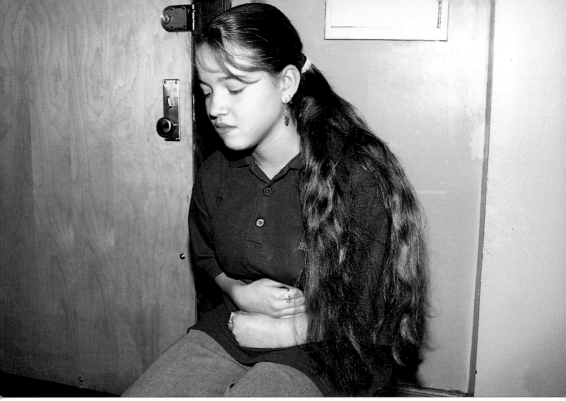

If symptoms such as fever, loss of appetite, weakness, and abdominal pains persist, you should schedule an appointment with a doctor to see if you have mononucleosis.

persist, you may have mononucleosis. Then it is time to see your doctor.

Fever. If you have a fever, keep a record of your temperature. If you're sick, you should tell your parents. They will know how to make you feel better. They may give you acetaminophen, such as Tylenol, or ibuprofen, such as Advil, to reduce your fever. Do not use aspirin, which has been known to cause Reye's syndrome in children and teenagers. This is a dangerous disorder that can be fatal.

Dehydration. Drink lots of liquids, such as water and juice, to prevent dehydration. Stay away from products that contain caffeine, such as coffee, tea, and soda. They can further dehydrate your body.

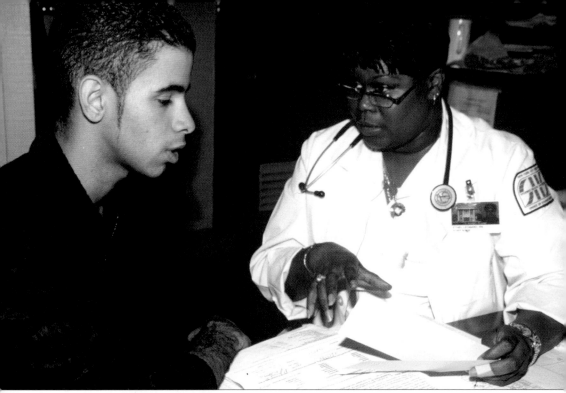

Only a doctor can determine whether you really have mononucleosis by giving you an examination and a blood test.

Fatigue. Get plenty of rest. Eat healthful foods. Try not to become stressed about your problems. Or better yet, try to avoid situations that you know will stress you out.

Runny nose. Try using a decongestant, but ask your parents or speak with a doctor about it first.

Sore throat. Gargle regularly with warm salt water. Lozenges can also be helpful to relieve a sore throat.

Loss of appetite. Try soups and breads, foods that are easy to snack on and are good for you. Eat plenty of fruit and vegetables. Eat at scheduled meal times even if you don't feel hungry. Your body needs the energy to function properly.

Nausea. Talk to your doctor about ways to feel better. Rest helps. So does drinking warm liquids, preferably decaffeinated teas. Products containing ginger, such as ginger ale, can help relieve nausea.

Swollen glands. Keep checking the glands at the sides of your neck (under your ears), or at the back of your knees and elbows, or on either side of your pelvis. If they're swollen and feel lumpy, you should schedule an appointment with your doctor. This is often indicative of something serious.

If these symptoms persist, see your doctor. He or she will examine you and give you a blood test. This is the only sure way to determine whether or not you have mononucleosis.

Other Symptoms

Other symptoms may also indicate that you have mononucleosis:

- persistent fever
- difficulty eating or drinking
- weakness
- persistent abdominal pains

If you are having abdominal pains, it is important to avoid injuring that area. The pain is the result of the spleen and liver working hard to filter out illness from the blood and the rest of the body. If you do have mononucleosis, you could rupture your spleen if you're not careful. It will be very sensitive during this time, while it works to fight the virus.

About 10 to 15 percent of mononucleosis sufferers have a skin rash. Ten percent may have jaundice. This is a liver condition that makes the eyes and skin look yellowish. Although it is rare, there are also people who experience problems with the heart, lungs, or spleen.

Doctor's Orders

If you do have mononucleosis, your doctor will tell you what you know already: There is little one can do to recover from mononucleosis besides getting plenty of rest. There are two stages in getting over mononucleosis. The first is getting over the symptoms. The second is making a full recovery.

Your doctor will offer suggestions about how to reduce your discomfort and treat your symptoms. Such suggestions are discussed in the next chapter.

In addition, your doctor will warn you about the need to take it easy even after your symptoms have disappeared. The disappearance of symptoms does not indicate a full recovery. The reason for this is discussed in detail in chapter 3.

Feeling Drained and Confused

According to people like Annie and Rosa, the worst part about having mononucleosis is the length of time it takes to recover. Patience and stamina are needed to keep from letting the disease depress you.

Other teens who have had mononucleosis say that the worst part about having the disease is wondering whether it is in their mind or in their body.

Teens suffering from mono are often concerned about this question. Unlike other childhood illnesses, such as chicken pox or the mumps, mononucleosis takes a long time to go away. It takes several weeks to work its way through the body. It can then take several months to get the body back to normal.

Also, mononucleosis doesn't have visible symptoms, except in rare cases of rashes and jaundice. You don't look sick. Some teens who have mononucleosis worry that they are not really sick, but are just imagining it. An examination by a doctor and a simple blood test are all that is needed to confirm that it really is mononucleosis.

Am I Contagious?

The time between your exposure to the Epstein-Barr virus and your first symptoms of mononucleosis is forty to fifty days. Whether the virus makes you sick or not depends on two things. First, did you have mono when you were a child? Second, in what condition were your immune and other systems at the time you were exposed to the virus? A weakened immune system may not be able to protect you against the virus whereas a healthy and strong body has a better chance of fighting off the virus.

The incubation period is the time between when a person becomes infected and when the symptoms first begin to show. This is also the most contagious period. Most people don't know they have mono until the symptoms show. During this time, they may have passed the virus to others.

By the time a person shows symptoms of mononucleosis, he or she is far less contagious, although care should still be taken not to infect anyone else. Avoid activities in which bodily fluids may be exchanged, such as kissing.

Chapter 3

How Do I Treat Mononucleosis?

Once your doctor has confirmed that you have mononucleosis, it is important to learn how to take care of yourself. Your doctor will tell you things you should do to help your body recover faster. He or she will also tell you what activities you should not do to avoid hindering your body's recovery process.

Getting Through It

People who have contracted mono catch it in different ways, but almost all agree that it is very uncomfortable once a person has it. Some teens with relatively mild cases continue going to school and doing other activities. But, more often than not, these teens also end up feeling even more tired than they would have if they had slowed down and rested. Some cases are so mild that the teens never realize they have mono.

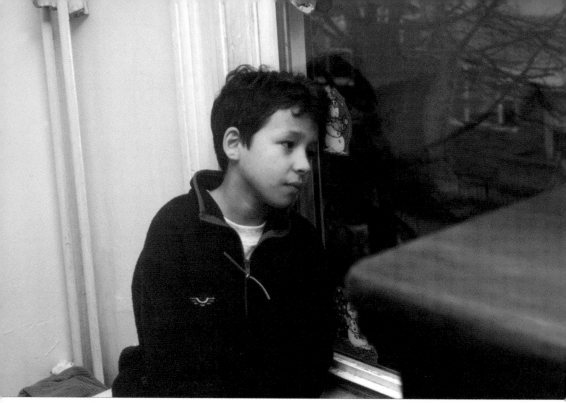

Recovering from mononucleosis requires lots of rest. Staying home instead of having fun with friends can be frustrating.

They may attribute their symptoms to stress, a cold, or the flu.

While it is not dangerous to be unaware that you have mono, it can be troublesome. This is because it can take you longer to return to your normal routine since you don't know you have to rest and stay in bed. No matter how mild a case of mono, the body still needs time and rest to properly recover. Without rest, the body takes longer to recover.

Others may have more severe cases and find that they feel terrible and must stay home until the mono runs its course through the body. These teens often feel extremely bored and fatigued. Even simple, everyday routines in their lives become a great effort. Activities such as combing their hair, brushing their teeth, or just getting out of bed can be draining.

Debra

When Debra contracted mono she thought she had the flu. She stayed home and rested and she felt better, but a week later she seemed to have the flu again. This pattern of having the flu over and over again continued until Debra concluded she must have a very bad illness. But her mother was very busy working all the time. Debra didn't want to worry her, so she didn't tell anyone about it.

As time went on, the symptoms started to become a real nuisance. Debra found herself feeling tired and temperamental. Everyday, she woke up feeling tired, fed herself feeling tired, went to school feeling tired, and did her chores feeling almost impossibly tired. Finally after six months, she began to feel like herself again.

It wasn't until several years later, long after Debra had recovered, that she even realized she had had mononucleosis. Debra says it changed her life because it made her realize how important it was for her to take care of herself properly. Eating a well-balanced diet, getting enough rest, and exercising help keep her body strong and healthy. She also says that if she had to do it all over again, she would definitely get a checkup with her doctor as soon as any symptoms appeared.

The Psychology of Getting Better

Doctors agree that the speed at which a person recovers

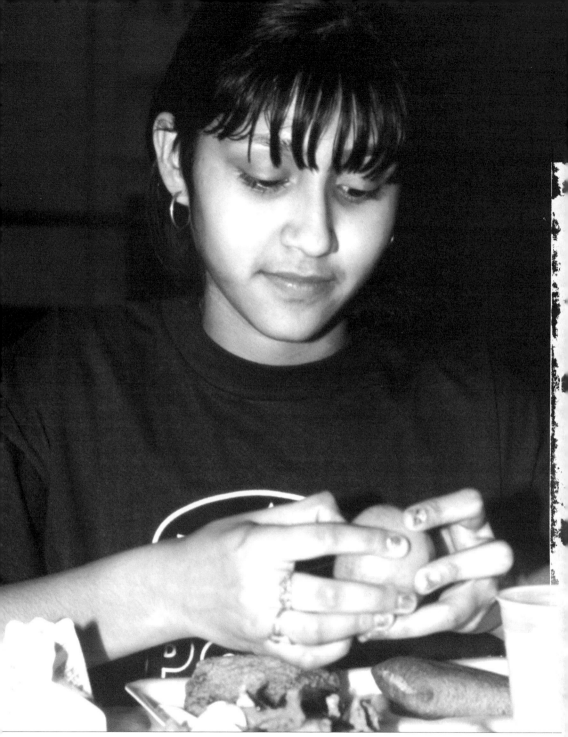

Eating healthful foods, such as fruits and vegetables, gives your body the nutrients and energy it needs to recover from mononucleosis.

from mononucleosis, or any major disease, is heavily influenced by his or her frame of mind. The more strongly motivated you are to get well, the faster your body is able to fight disease. The more depressed you are, the longer you tend to stay sick.

It is true that you are more susceptible to other diseases after you have battled another, because your immune system may have been weakened by fighting the other illness. Thinking positively and focusing your energy on getting well may help your immune system grow stronger.

Getting Over the Symptoms

In addition to trying to keep an upbeat attitude, it is important to rest your body. Most doctors order their patients to cut down on their activities for at least a month, until their symptoms disappear, and to keep their schedules light and easy for another month after that.

Most teens may become easily frustrated and bored during this time. Many teens lead active lives. They are occupied with school and homework, as well as extracurricular activities. There are also parties to go to and friends to hang out with. Most teens like to keep busy. But when teens get mono, they are no longer able to do any of their normal activities. This can be quite a shock, and some teens may have a hard time coping with it. Their friends are out having fun, while they are stuck home in bed. This one thought alone can be

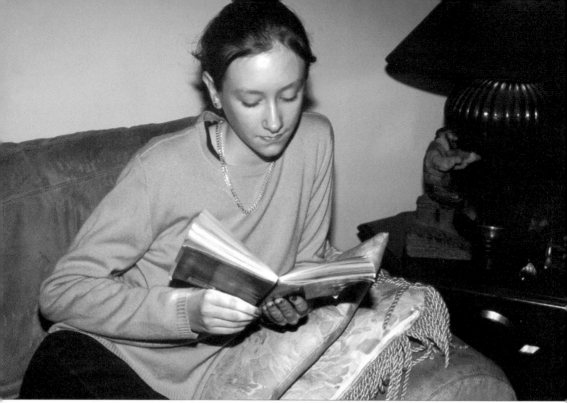
Some teens who have mononucleosis occupy their time by reading books by their favorite authors.

enough to depress some teens. Fortunately, there are things you can do to make yourself more comfortable and make the time pass more quickly.

Practice perseverance. The first thing is to practice perseverance. This means being patient, which can be hard, especially for teens. Remind yourself that time is working for you, not against you. Take everything one day at a time. Don't think about how many more days you have to stay in bed. Think instead that every day that you spend in bed, you are giving your body the time it needs to recover.

Drink fluids. Drink a lot of liquids, especially water and juice, or soup. Normally you should drink about eight glasses of water each day, so increase your intake.

This will keep your body from becoming dehydrated and will also help flush the illness out of your system.

Take vitamins. Vitamins C and E and the mineral zinc are all good for your immune system. Your doctor may recommend these or other vitamins. Take them as directed by your doctor.

Eat well. Eat the right kinds of foods—a balanced diet with protein, breads and grains, dairy products, fruits, and vegetables. Your body needs these foods to fuel the work it needs to do to repair itself. Your doctor may also be able to recommend special foods that your body needs. Try to stay away from junk food, such as candy and chips. These foods often have no nutritional value. The high counts of salt and sugar normally found in these foods can make you feel worse.

Sleep well. Sleep is one of the most important things you can do for your body. While you sleep, your body focuses all of its energy on getting well. Sleep as much as you can. Don't feel guilty about taking naps. Sleeping is also the best way to pass time.

Communicate. You may find that some people are not knowledgeable about your disease. They may make false assumptions about you and the disease. If you find that these assumptions are hurtful, help them better understand the disease by giving them facts to dispel the false ideas.

The Recovery Process
Keep your spirits up. First, keep yourself as busy as

you can. If you can't concentrate enough to read, look at books with beautiful images. Try listening to an audiobook, a book on tape. If you're watching television, try skipping the commercials by hitting the mute button or changing channels. Commercials are usually louder and more stress-inducing than the programs. Or you can ask your parents to rent you some of your favorite movies.

Second, try something new but nonstressful. Try watching longer movies that have an easy pace instead of action-packed films. Listen to a wider range of music. Try using your time of required rest to learn about classical music, jazz, or some other type of music.

Third, keep yourself occupied. Try drawing some pictures. Daydream. Talk on the telephone for as long as you can. But don't talk so long that you become resentful of what's going on in the outside world while you're in bed, or mad that someone's not being understanding. The trick is to maintain your enthusiasm, your connection to the world you will eventually be returning to.

Be gentle with yourself. Take good care of your body, but there is no need to baby yourself. Be careful of your stomach area. Avoid doing anything strenuous that risks bursting your spleen. And be careful about catching any other illnesses while your immune system is busy battling mono.

If you have allergies, try to stay away from things that may cause you to have an allergic reaction. Also, don't go near people who have the flu or a cold. Your weakened immune system may not be able to fight the germs off.

Can I Contract Mononucleosis Again?

Except for extremely rare cases, a person contracts mononucleosis only once. However, problems or weaknesses with your immune system and the Epstein-Barr virus can recur later in life if you don't take care of yourself. Chronic fatigue syndrome (CFS), which has many symptoms similar to mono, is a newly diagnosed disease that can affect you later in life. This is a condition that affects mostly adults. Doctors are currently studying it to find ways to treat it.

Chronic Fatigue Syndrome

CFS has symptoms very similar to those of mononucleosis. People with CFS feel very tired all the time and are unable to concentrate. Many experience trouble sleeping. Other symptoms include mild fevers, muscle pain, sore throats, and swollen lymph glands.

Adults, who appear to be beyond the age of contracting mononucleosis, tend to be the ones who contract CFS. People who have CFS become too tired to continue more than half their usual workload. This frequently leads to depression, which may undercut the body's ability to fight off the disease.

CFS is not a form of mononucleosis, but because the symptoms of the two illnesses are so similar, doctors

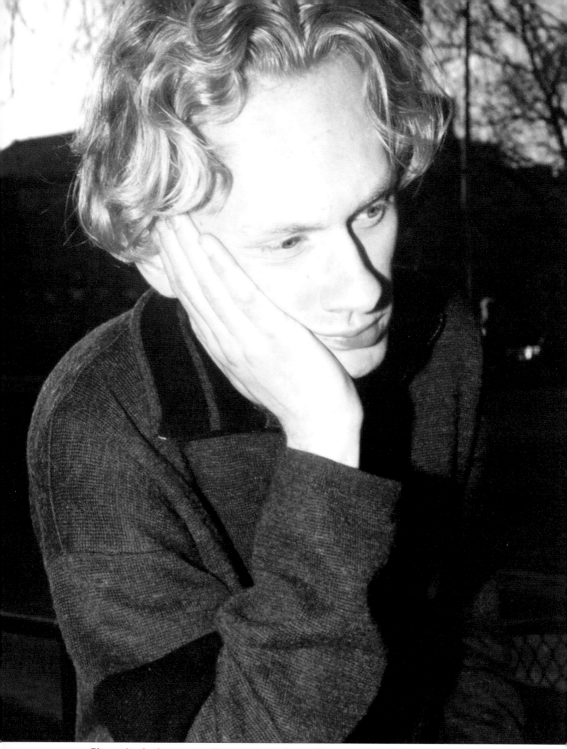
Chronic fatigue syndrome (CFS) is a disease that has symptoms similar to mononucleosis, such as fatigue and depression.

may mistakenly give a diagnosis of mono when it is really CFS. Tests conducted on CFS patients indicate a positive presence of the Epstein-Barr virus in some people but a negative presence in others. At the same time, doctors have also noted that some people who have had mononucleosis also get CFS. There may be a connection between the two illnesses that scientists have not yet identified.

Chapter 4

Full Recovery Takes Time

*C*hris was a high school football player. He felt mildly ill for a few weeks, but he didn't think it was anything serious. But when he didn't start to feel better, he finally went to see his doctor. The doctor ran some tests and determined that Chris had mononucleosis. For Chris, one of the worst results of mono was that he could no longer play the sport he loved. It was his first season as a starter. He couldn't believe how unfair it was that he couldn't play football. This depressed him.

He soon grew too tired even to see his girlfriend. He felt too tired and depressed to even talk to her on the telephone. He also grew depressed thinking of how all his friends were out having a great time and he was stuck in bed. He grew bored watching television and tired of being at home all the time. But he was also far too tired to go out. He couldn't wait until he was over the disease, which seemed to be taking forever.

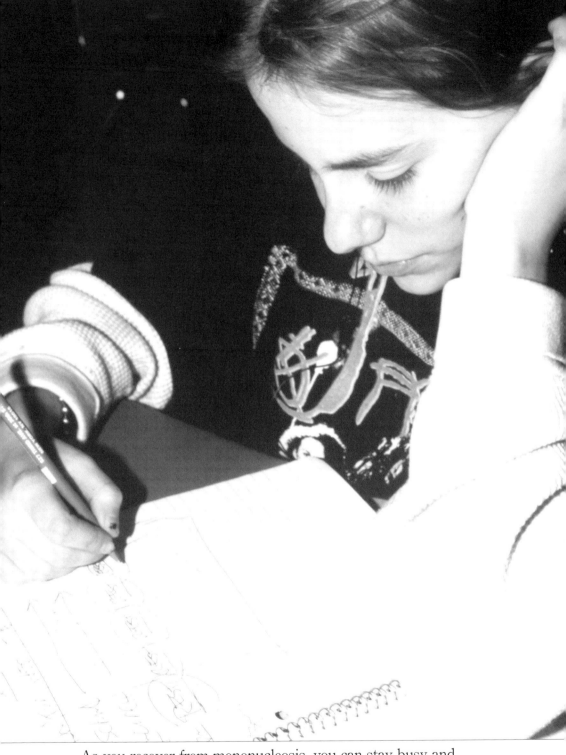

As you recover from mononucleosis, you can stay busy and keep your spirits up by drawing, writing, or listening to music.

Getting Better

Get regular checkups from your doctor so you will know when you're really doing better, and what you should do then. Most of what your doctor says will seem simple—take it easy, eat and drink well. It is important that your doctor also keep track of you so those rare complications, such as skin rashes, jaundice, or heart, lung, or abdominal problems don't occur. Your doctor will check you for all of those symptoms. He or she will feel your abdomen and will tell you how you are doing and how far you still have to go.

You will get through a month of painful swollen glands, constant sore throats, stomachaches, fevers, headaches, and being constantly tired. Gradually, however, you will start getting out to do little things so you will not be depressed. During this time at home, you may even have learned to like some new books, films, or music. You will have learned about patience and perseverance. Most of your symptoms will have disappeared, and you will begin to feel better.

Now comes the tricky part. You feel good enough to take up your old routine. You may be impatient to get out and do things you haven't been able to do for a month. But your doctor tells you that you need to keep an easy pace for another month. You ask, "Why?"

Avoid a Relapse

Earlier, we learned about Rosa and Debra and their bouts with mono. Rosa ended up having the disease all summer, a total of nearly four months. Why did it take her so long to recover? Partly it was her depression at missing out on summer vacation. Partly it was the length of time her body needed to battle the Epstein-Barr virus.

Rosa

When Rosa finally started getting out to do things again, her doctor cautioned her to keep taking it easy. He told her that if she didn't, she could end up with a relapse. A relapse is when a disease comes back for a second time, instead of disappearing from the body, the way colds often do. It takes longer to recover from a relapse of mononucleosis than to get over the initial bout of illness.

Since Rosa had taken four months to feel better, she paid attention to her doctor's advice. She didn't resume her normal schedule until nearly Christmas. And by then she had picked up some new healthy habits along the way. She took vitamins every day, exercised regularly, and learned to eat well-balanced meals and drink lots of fluids.

Debra

Debra recovered from her initial bout with mononucleosis in four weeks. But since she never knew she had mono because she never saw a doctor, she returned to her normal schedule too soon after getting over her symptoms. After being cooped up at home, she tried to

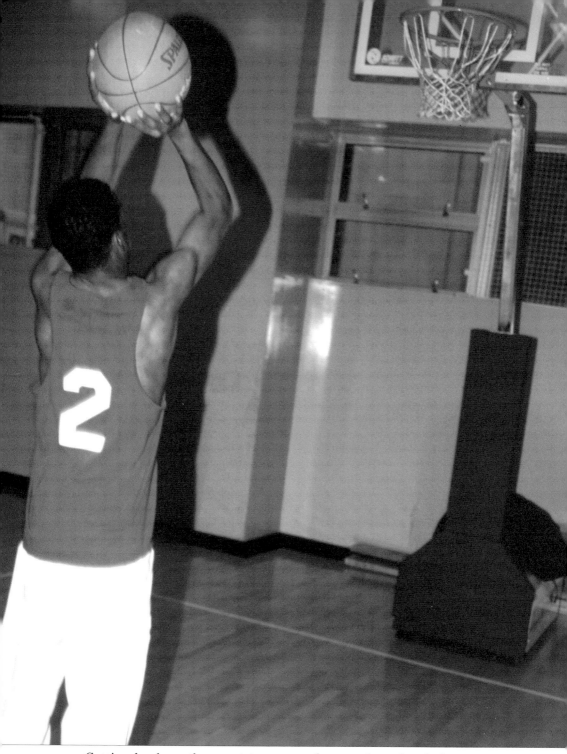

Getting back on the court too soon after you have battled mononucleosis is risky because you could suffer a relapse.

make up for lost fun by spending more and more time than ever outside. The activities pushed her body physically further than it was prepared for.

Within a month of "getting better," she caught what she thought was the flu again and had to stay in bed for a week. This made her depressed, and the week stretched into two.

It was nearly a year before the cycle of busy periods and a recurring "flu" worked themselves out. It was only later that Debra realized that she had had mononucleosis.

Chris

Chris recovered from his symptoms within a couple of months. He had listened to his doctor's advice about attitude and rest. He also found activities that occupied his time and that didn't tire him easily while at home in bed. Although Chris missed the football season, he kept up his spirits by thinking to himself that basketball season was just around the corner.

By the start of Christmas vacation, Chris was beginning to feel like himself again. He was glad that he would have a couple of weeks of vacation to get back in shape before basketball practice started.

Allow Your Entire Body to Heal

Doctors generally tell patients to wait a month or longer after symptoms have disappeared before going back to their normal routines. This means patients should not engage in strenuous activities or they risk the possibility of a relapse.

One result of your body's fight with an infectious viral disease like mononucleosis is that the virus continues to affect the immune system even after all the symptoms have disappeared.

In other words, once your symptoms are gone you will start to get your energy back. You will stop running fevers. Your sore throat will go away, and your painfully swollen glands will return to normal. But your body's great battlegrounds—your spleen, thymus, tonsils, and lymph systems—will stay enlarged for some time after the rest of your body recovers. That is why it is important to maintain a light schedule for at least a month after your symptoms have disappeared. The danger is that, because you start feeling better, you may overdo activities while your body is still weak.

Chris took care of himself well throughout the first weeks of recovery. He took vitamins, drank fluids, and ate well-balanced meals. By Christmas time his symptoms were gone.

A few days after Christmas, Chris went to the basketball courts outside his school to shoot a few hoops. He planned to take it easy. He started out just standing in one place, shooting, and walking to get the ball. Then he started retrieving the ball more actively and kept moving to a new spot to shoot. He tried a few rebounds. When some friends came and suggested that he join them in

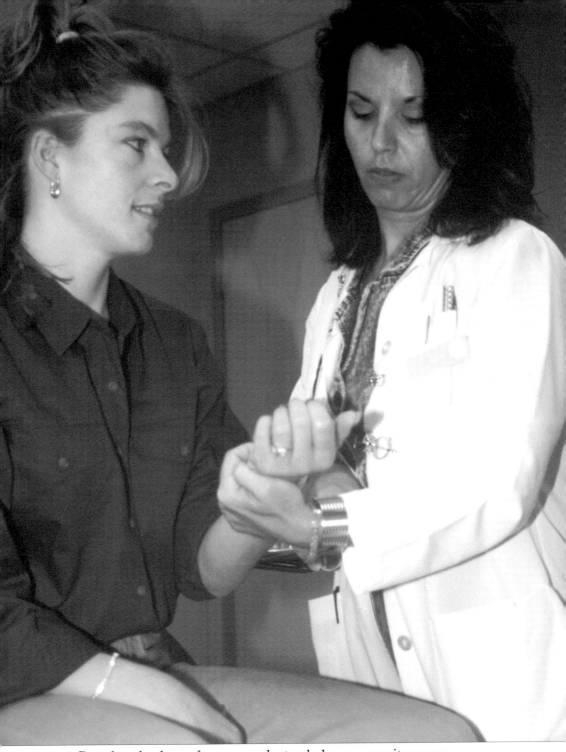

Regular checkups from your doctor help you monitor your recovery from mononucleosis.

a quick pick-up game, Chris said no. He just wasn't well enough. He kept on shooting.

All of a sudden Chris found himself in incredible pain. He was rushed to the nearest hospital. There the doctor found that Chris's spleen, enlarged and tender as it was from battling mononucleosis, had come close to rupturing.

A Close Call

Chris's doctor explained what had happened to his spleen. The spleen destroys sick blood cells in the body. It also filters and stores blood. It is located in the upper abdomen, under the ribs. When fighting mono, the spleen, along with the thymus, tonsils, and other lymph nodes, enlarge three to four times normal size because they have so much work to do. This is what causes the pain involved with mono.

When Chris was shooting hoops, he pushed his body too far. It had not had enough time to recover completely. His spleen was still enlarged. As a result of the physical activity, his spleen nearly split open.

Fortunately, a rupture was averted. Chris had to stay in bed for a full week and a half. He also had to stop most physical activity for several months. Doctors worked to drain his enlarged spleen. He suffered severe abdominal pains and nosebleeds for close to a month. In the end, he had to take it easy into the next fall. This time, his doctor and parents made certain he fully recuperated before he started any strenuous activities.

Little by Little

As Chris could tell you, once you have recovered from the symptoms of mononucleosis, take the time to let your body heal completely. Give yourself at least one month of rest before starting strenuous physical activity. If you exercise or play a sport, start slowly and be sure you get your physician's approval. Keep eating well. Stay away from sweets and junk food, which can weaken the body. Take vitamins, especially vitamin C. Get plenty of sleep. Practice the many lessons about taking care of yourself that you learned while getting through the disease itself.

Chapter 5

Protecting Yourself

Mononucleosis is not a life-threatening condition, but it can cause a great deal of discomfort and disruption in the lives of the people who contract this disease.

An Ounce of Prevention

The only way you can try to prevent contracting mononucleosis is to take care of yourself. Get a lot of sleep. Don't let stress wear you down. Eat well. Take vitamins. Keep your body and immune system strong by engaging in physical activities, such as walking, jogging, or school sports. Be careful about whom you kiss. As this disease can be passed through sexual activities, if you are going to have sex, be sure of your partner's sexual history. Always use a condom. Have regular checkups with your doctor.

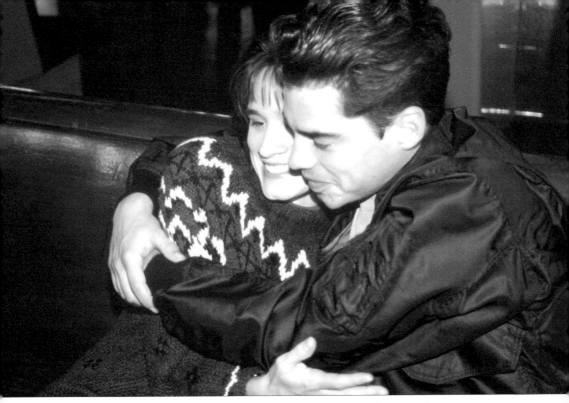

Since mononucleosis can be transmitted through sexual contact, it's important to protect yourself by practicing safe sex.

Although stress is a part of everyone's life, it can be managed. Take time to free yourself of stress. Exercise helps rid the body of stress. Keeping a journal, too, can help you understand what you are feeling and can help you reduce stress. Talk with friends or a trusted adult if something is worrying you. Make certain you get enough sleep. And, if you find you have too many activities jammed into your schedule, think about which of them you might be able to cut out of your schedule for a while.

Stress of the Teen Years

Life as a young adult isn't easy. It is a time when you suddenly have to make lots of decisions on your own,

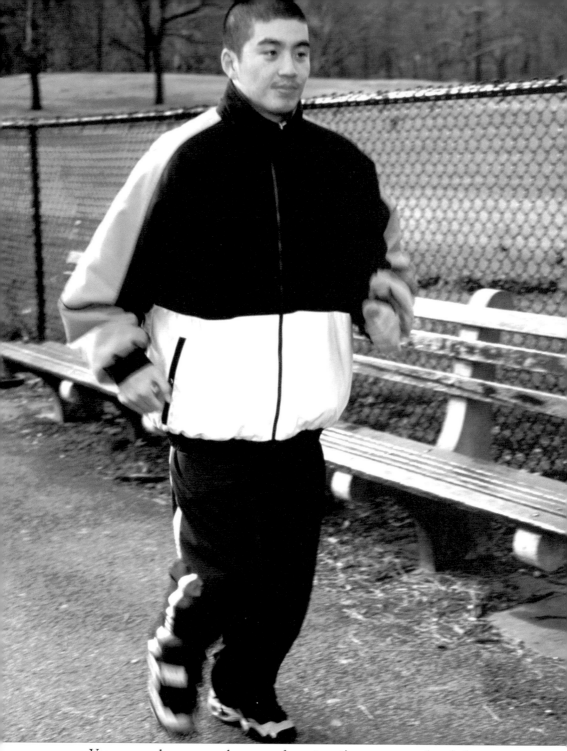

You can reduce your chances of contracting mononucleosis by exercising regularly, which keeps your immune system strong.

but in many cases you are still treated like a kid by some of the adults in your life. You may also face pressure from your friends or classmates about certain aspects of your life, such as how you dress and whom you date. There is also the pressure that comes from your changing body and ideas as you mature and learn more about life and yourself. This leads to stress on three levels—with your peers, with adults, and within yourself.

Regaining Health

If you do contract mononucleosis, slow down. See your doctor, and take time to recover completely. For many teenagers, the big hurdles to overcome are depression and impatience. Your body moves less quickly than your brain. Your body will naturally recover from mononucleosis, if you give it the rest it needs. But this process of recovery takes time. Even if your brain tells you that you can go back to your normal routine, your body isn't ready. It may be difficult, but the only way you can fully recover from mono is to give your body the time it needs to heal properly. Treat your body well. Maintain good health habits.

Good health is directly related to good attitudes. If you contract mononucleosis, find ways to keep yourself from being bored. By keeping busy, you are less likely to become depressed, and this will help your body recover faster.

Once your symptoms are gone, remember to allow yourself at least one more month to recover. During that period, do not do any strenuous physical activity.

Taking the time to recover will help you avoid a relapse or a worsening of your condition.

Annie, Rosa, Debra, and Chris learned, by dealing with mononucleosis, that their bodies have powerful ways of fighting illness. They learned what they can do to help their body fight illness. They also learned to be patient and to persevere.

Your body, too, has many ways to protect itself from illness and disease. But even if you do get sick, your body will eventually be able to recover. Be patient and give your body the time it needs to recover fully. An illness like mononucleosis with its long recovery process may seem unbearable, but it will pass. You will get through it. And you will learn valuable lessons about yourself along the way.

Glossary

chronic fatigue syndrome A disease that causes symptoms similar to mononucleosis. This disease usually affects adults.

contagious Something, such as a cold, that can be spread unknowingly through contact.

dehydration Process in which the body is not getting enough fluids.

diagnosis Identifying an illness or disease through tests and examination.

Epstein-Barr virus The virus that causes mononucleosis.

fatigue An extreme feeling of tiredness.

herpes virus A contagious virus passed on through saliva that causes diseases such as chicken pox, mumps, fever blisters, cold sores, and mono. Another variation of this virus can also cause a sexually transmitted disease.

immune system A system that protects the body from bacteria, viruses, and other invading germs.

infectious Disease or illness spread by infection.

jaundice A liver condition that causes symptoms including yellowish eyes and skin.

liver An organ in the body that filters impurities from the blood and is the body's main cleansing unit.

lymphatic system The main part of the body's immune system; it serves to filter all fluids in the body.

perseverance Sticking to a goal or purpose without giving up or faltering.

relapse To fall or slip back into a previous condition.

rupture The tearing apart of a tissue or an organ.

spleen The organ that produces cells that clean the blood.

tonsils Two small, oval-shaped membranes found in the sides of the throat that filter out impurities that pass through the mouth.

viruses Infective agents that invade the body cells and cause serious diseases.

Where to Go for Help

The best sources for help for mononucleosis are your parents, doctor, or school nurse. You can also look in your local Yellow Pages for the number of your state health department. Below are sources for information about mononucleosis.

American Medical Association
Headquarters
515 North State St.
Chicago, IL 60610
312-464-5000
Web site: http://www.ama-assn.org/

Centers for Disease Control and Prevention (CDC)
1600 Clifton Rd. NE
Atlanta, GA 30333
404-639-3311
Web site: http://www.cdc.gov/

National Institutes of Health
National Institute of Allergy and Infectious Diseases
Office of Communications
Building 31, Room 7A50
Bethesda, MD 20892
301-496-5717
Web site: http://www.nih.gov/

For Further Reading

Ayer, Eleanor H. *Everything You Need to Know About Depression.* Rev. ed. New York: The Rosen Publishing Group, 1997.

———. *Everything You Need to Know About Stress.* Rev. ed. New York: The Rosen Publishing Group. 1998.

Laurel, Shader, and John Zonerman. *Mononucleosis and Other Infectious Diseases.* New York: Chelsea House Publishing, 1989.

Martin, Ann M. *Get Well Soon, Mallory!* New York: Scholastic, Inc., 1993.

Silverstein, Alvin, Virginia Silverstein, and Robert Silverstein. *Mononucleosis.* Springfield, NJ: Enslow Publishing, 1994.

Stoffman, Phyllis. *The Family Guide to Preventing and Treating 100 Infectious Illnesses.* New York: John Wiley & Sons, 1995.

Index

About the Author

Paul Smart, a freelance writer of over twenty years, has been editing the Catskill Mountains leading weekly newspaper, *The Mountain Eagle*, in upstate New York. He is the author of local histories, screenplays, and poetry, in addition to ghostwriting nonfiction works on dentistry and music.

Photo Credits

Photos on pp. 18, 34 by Pablo Maldonado; All other photos by Ira Fox.